STOP HEART ATTACK NOW

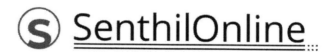

STOP
HEART
ATTACK
NOW!

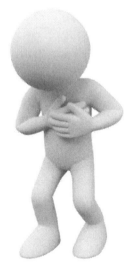

3 Step Formula
To Stop The Number One
Killer Of Men And Women
(1 Step Is Optional!)

SENTHIL NATARAJAN

Disclaimer

I am Not a Doctor or Medical Practitioner. Keep that in mind and please check with your cardiologist or your physician, licensed health provider or health care practitioner, if you have any questions about implementing any lifestyle changes mentioned in this book. You are fore-warned!

The information contained in this book is not intended to be a substitute for professional medical advice or treatment and is for educational purposes only. Results from following the information in this book will vary from individual to individual. If you have any health concerns or concerns about potential risks, you should always check with your physician, licensed health provider or health care practitioner.

The products and its description are not been evaluated by the food & drug administration (FDA). The products mentioned are not intended to diagnose, treat, cure or prevent any diseases.
Information on this book is not an alternative to medical advice from your doctor or other professional healthcare provider. Please consult your physician, or health care provider before taking any home remedies.

The ideas, procedures, and suggestions in this book are not intended as a substitute for consulting with a physician. All matters of health require medical supervision. The author shall be not be liable or responsible for any loss or damage allegedly arising from any information or suggestion in this book.

YOUR FREE BONUS

Dear reader, as a small token of thanks for buying this book, I'd like to offer you a free bonus gift exclusive to my readers.

I am offering a **FREE Series** called "Heart Health Drinks Series"...

Improve Your Heart Health Starting Today!

You can get the **FREE GIFT** by signing up here:

https://www.senthilonline.com/FREE/

Introduction

__"Health is wealth"__

The statistics on heart attack and heart diseases in the United States is shocking. See below:

Statistics on Heart Attack[1]

1. **In the United States, someone has a heart attack every 40 seconds.**

2. Every year, about 805,000 Americans have a heart attack. Of these, 605,000 are a first heart attack

3. 200,000 happen to people who have already had a heart attack

4. About 1 in 5 heart attacks is silent—the damage is done, but the person is not aware of it.

Statistics on Heart Disease[1]

1. **Heart disease is the leading cause of death for men, women, and people of most racial and ethnic groups in the United States.**

2. One person dies every 37 seconds in the United States from cardiovascular disease.

3. About 647,000 Americans die from heart disease each year—that's 1 in every 4 deaths.

4. Heart disease costs the United States about $219 billion each year from 2014 to 2015. This includes the cost of health care services, medicines, and lost productivity due to death.

I suffered from a heart attack, went through surgery and a recovery process. I wanted to share what I learnt in these few years about heart health.

Though I kept postponing writing a book, whenever I saw and heard news about people dying of heart disease like heart attack etc., it really pained me. Research shows it need not be that way.

In fact, research shows heart disease can even be reversed! [2]

Over the past three years I learnt many things related to heart health. Tidbits of information I gathered, applied and benefitted for heart health and for my overall health.

I wanted to share this information to a wider audience, so anyone could have a good understanding of heart health in less than a few hours and can implement the things I mention in this book.

I honestly wish no one should go through the pain of heart diseases, surgery etc.

And You Can Do It!

If you just follow the 3 simple steps provided int this book. I wish you achieve a healthy heart in a natural way by following information provided in this book.

And if you did that, it's a favor, you did for yourself, your family and friends and to the society in general.

Wishing everyone a healthy heart and good health!
Senthil Natarajan

Note: My research on various topics in this book led to various sources that provided heart health videos, scientific proof, what to eat, what to do for overall heart health etc., I have provided these links wherever I referred to or used them.

Since there were many sources, I have included a section called "Links and References". Here you will find all the links mentioned in this book in one place. It should be handy for you.

How to get the best out of this book?

To get the best out of this book, please go through all the links, including the video links in this book. You'll learn a lot about heart health and overall health in a short time. So, please use it.

Source[1]:
https://www.cdc.gov/heartdisease/facts.htm

Source[2]: Prevent and Reverse Heart Disease by Caldwell B. Esselstyn, Jr., MD – Various angiograms on Reversal of Coronary Disease.

Check my review for this book at:
https://www.senthilonline.com/prevent-and-reverse-heart-disease/

To my wife & son

Table Of Contents

1.My Story

"Prevention is better than cure"

1.1 Day Of Attack

Saturday, April 1, 2017. It started as any other weekend for me. I did not have any plans on that day. Around 10:00AM in the morning, suddenly I felt heaviness in my chest and I couldn't breathe. I went to the balcony to get more air. Still I was not able to breathe normally.

I didn't realize the severity of the situation and decided to go to the urgent care nearby instead of calling 911 or going to emergency!

It was a long wait in the urgent care center. After more than an hour I was called in. I explained what I was going through. To relieve my breathlessness, I was provided an inhaler and was asked to inhale it. I don't remember the exact medication now.

I was also provided a nitroglycerin medicine to relieve my chest pain. My blood pressure came down rapidly after that. The nurse asked me to take rest, for the rest of the day.

We came back late in the afternoon to home. And in the evening, we went to the pharmacy to get our medication. I did not feel good at the time and sat on the floor there. Someone even asked me if I was okay. We reached around 11.00 PM at night. I took some prescription medicine and went to sleep.

But instead of going to sleep, it seems I said something and was about to slip into an unconscious state. My wife shook me up and she was terrified. I consoled her and she stayed with me the whole night.

Sunday, I did not go anywhere. I was just taking a rest. I could still feel a heaviness in my heart. One of my friends called me in the evening and asked how I was. I told him I was having chest pains. When he asked how I was feeling, I said it was like an elephant sitting on my chest. Really, I felt like that.

Monday, my wife was searching for a primary care physician (we had moved in recently) and we found one near our home. We met our primary care physician. I told my symptoms and the chest pain issue I had that weekend.

The doctor immediately performed an ECG (Electrocardiogram) on me. And after seeing the results, he referred me to a cardiologist and said I should see him right away.

I drove to the cardiologist office and the doctor was already briefed by my primary care physician at that time. He too did an ECG on me and then asked me to get admitted to the Hospital immediately. The hospital was thankfully just 5 minutes away.

We went to the hospital emergency room and I got myself admitted there. In the hospital they did one more ECG. I asked the nurse to show me the result. The ECG graph was not normal per nurse.

The nurse gave me the patient dress and asked me to wear it. After that, I was asked to sit on a wheel-chair and she took me to the operation theater. While I was in a wheelchair, 4 to 5 nurses came. They injected something on me and they were rushing me to the operation theater.

In the operation theater, I saw my cardiologist who I met before. I was somewhat relieved to see someone I knew of, even though I had just met him. The last thing I remember was that I was on the operating table and I was talking to my cardiologist.

Fast forward and one hour later, I woke up and saw many nurses, few doctors, my cardiologist around me. I was surprised to know they did surgery on me within an hour. I was told that they put a stent on one of my heart arteries.

I asked the doctor if they have to do this now. He said "Yes, we have to save you. You had a heart attack".

What is ECG or EKG?

ECG/EKG stands for Electrocardiogram. It is a test to check signs of heart disease. For more details about ECG/EKG check the following link.

Source:
https://www.webmd.com/heart-disease/electrocardiogram-ekgs#1

1.2 My Angioplasty Experience

1.2.1 What Is Angioplasty And Stenting?

I went through a procedure called angioplasty. Angioplasty opens narrowed coronary arteries in the heart using stents. A good explanation is provided in the video below, courtesy Mayo Clinic.

https://www.mayoclinic.org/tests-procedures/coronary-angioplasty/multimedia/coronary-angioplasty/vid-20084728

In case if you cannot access the above video, check the video below.

https://www.youtube.com/watch?v=S9AqBd4R Exk

1.2.2 Stent

A wire mesh tube that holds open weakened remove and arteries. The stent may prevent re-narrowing after an artery has widened and it stays in place permanently as the blood vessel lining heals over it.

1.2.3 Details About My Angioplasty

My angioplasty was done using the femoral artery in the groin. A stent was placed in my Right Coronary Artery (RCA).

After the procedure, I was feeling pain in the groin area. I suffered from bleeding after the procedure. My cardiologist informed my wife that I may have to go for blood transfusion, if it won't stop. It is really a painful situation for any spouse to undergo this experience.

Thankfully my bleeding stopped after sometime. I had to lie flat for a number of hours for the next few days. When I started walking after it healed, I could only walk very slowly, taking baby steps.

I kept my palm over the groin area when I walked. Because you have to be careful for a few days before the blood vessel heals.

1.3 Challenges After Discharge From Hospital

The following are the two major challenges I faced after being discharged from the hospital.

1.   Pain in the groin area and
2.   Going to sleep with this pain

1.3.1 How To Overcome Groin Pain When Lying Flat?

One thing that nobody tells you, if your angioplasty procedure is done in the groin area is, the pain that you have to undergo for some time until the wound heals.

In hospital they provide you with a folding bed and you rest and sleep on it. Because of the folding bed, you don't experience much pain while you are in the hospital. Since you don't lie flat when you sleep, you won't feel that much pain in the groin area when you sleep.

If you have a folding bed in your home then I think you will not suffer much. Since I had only regular bed at home, it was really painful when you try to sleep flatly on it and when you try to get up from the bed. I have to be ingenious and find some solution.

I stacked a bunch of pillows and tried my best so that I won't lie flat and somewhat managed this issue. I wish somebody told me this beforehand.

1.3.2 How To Get To Sleep With Groin Pain?

If you are having difficulty sleeping with pain, I would suggest you listen to whatever makes you sleep. The trick is to listen to something repetitive. Remember the lullaby songs that you heard when you were a baby. I found listening to chants helped me get to sleep quicker.

1.3.3 Isha Chants App Links

I used the following chant app from Isha Chants. They have many chants. Choose the one you like. Before you sleep, select a mantra or song and just listen... until you fall asleep.

My favorite chants in Isha Chants app are, "Shambo" and "Brahmananda Swaroopa" chants.

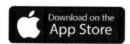

https://apps.apple.com/us/app/isha-chants/id1158670101

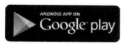

https://play.google.com/store/apps/details?id=org.ishafoundation.app.chants&hl=en_US

1.4 Lifestyle change - My Eureka Moment!

After discharge from the hospital, I went for my first blood work on June 30th 2017. You can see the lipid panel results below. You can see I had a high triglyceride count of 221.

Order Date: 06/30/2017   Received: 07/01/2017 04:10:07

Collection Date: 06/30/2017 12:32:00   Report: 07/01/2017 03:47:00

LIPID PANEL

	NAME	VALUE	REFERENCE RANGE
F	CHOLESTEROL, TOTAL	112 L	125-200 (mg/dL)
F	HDL CHOLESTEROL	32 L	> OR = 40 (mg/dL)
F	TRIGLYCERIDES	221 H	<150 (mg/dL)
F	LDL-CHOLESTEROL	36	<130 (mg/dL (calc))

1.4.1 What Are Triglycerides?

Medicineplus says "Triglycerides are a type of fat. They are the most common type of fat in your body. They come from foods, especially butter, oils, and other fats you eat. Triglycerides also come from extra calories.

These are the calories that you eat, but your body does not need right away. Your body changes these extra calories into triglycerides, and stores them in fat cells.

When your body needs energy, it releases the triglycerides. Having a high level of triglycerides can raise your risk of heart diseases, such as coronary artery disease."

Source:
https://medlineplus.gov/triglycerides.html

Since I had a high triglyceride count, I wanted to reduce this. I was already under statins and I did not want to take more medicines to reduce side effects. I was discussing with doctor and nurse about other alternatives to reduce my triglyceride counts.

One of the items in the discussion was about my food habits. After knowing that I ate white rice the nurse suggested that I switch to brown rice. All my life I was eating polished white rice.

I did not think much about changing from white rice to brown rice. I just went to the store and bought a bag of organic brown rice and started eating it for lunch only from that day onwards.

Around four months later I went for another blood work. Boy...was I surprised! You can see the results below.

Accession ID: BA831018A

Lab Ref ID: 0009075

Order Date: 10/27/2017

Received: 11/02/2017 08:49:35

Collection Date: 10/27/2017 10:44:00

Report: 10/28/2017 02:53:00

LIPID PANEL

	NAME	VALUE	REFERENCE RANGE
F	CHOLESTEROL, TOTAL	89	<200 (mg/dL)
F	**HDL CHOLESTEROL**	31 L	>40 (mg/dL)
F	TRIGLYCERIDES	77	<150 (mg/dL)
F	LDL-CHOLESTEROL	42	(mg/dL (calc))

My triglycerides decreased from 221 to 77! **A 65% reduction in 4 months, just by making a simple change.** By quitting eating polished white rice and start eating organic brown rice. How hard was it?

This was the eureka moment! If by making a small dietary change, I could reduce my excess triglyceride level, what else I can do to save my heart and overall health.

The following chapters are some of my answers to that question. Before we try to solve a problem, I think it's wise to know about the problem. Right?

Let's understand the problem "What Heart Attack is?" in simple terms in the next chapter.

Disclosure: I was also taking statins during this time. My most recent lab results show triglycerides count of 115 after reducing statin intake to 5mg per day. Now I am out of statins.

2.What is a Heart Attack?

"A problem well stated is a problem half-solved".

-Charles Kettering

Before I tell you what a heart attack is, it is important to understand the following:

1. Heart
2. Plaque and
3. Coronary Artery Disease (CAD)

2.1 Heart

Let's understand the heart. The first thing to know is that the **heart is a powerful muscular organ** responsible for pumping blood through arteries and veins.

Arteries and Veins are both blood vessels. Arteries carry oxygen-rich blood away from the heart to the body and veins carry oxygen-poor blood from the body to the heart for re-oxygenation.

The heart itself needs oxygenated blood for heart muscles to work. If the heart muscles don't get oxygen rich blood, they die.

Let me repeat that sentence again - If the heart muscles don't get oxygen rich blood, they die. So, remember this.

2.2 What Is Plaque?[2.2]

Plaque is made up of deposits of cholesterol and other substances in the artery. Plaque buildup causes the inside of the arteries to narrow over time, which can partially or totally block the blood flow. This process is called atherosclerosis.

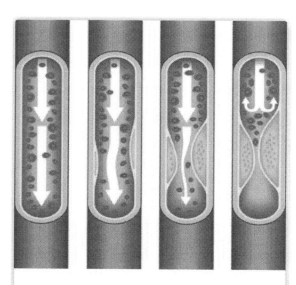

As plaque builds up in the arteries of a person with heart disease, the inside of the arteries begins to narrow, which lessens or blocks the flow of blood. Plaques can also rupture (break open) and when they do a blood clot can form on the plaque, blocking the flow of blood.

About Plaque, Picture Source and Caption[2.2]

Source:
https://www.cdc.gov/heartdisease/facts.htm

2.3 What Is Coronary Artery Disease?[2.3]

Coronary artery disease (CAD) is the most common type of heart disease in the United States. It is sometimes called coronary heart disease or ischemic heart disease.
For some people, the first sign of CAD is a heart attack. You and your health care team may be able to help reduce your risk for CAD.

What Causes Coronary Artery Disease?[2.3]

CAD is caused by plaque buildup in the walls of the arteries that supply blood to the heart (called coronary arteries) and other parts of the body.

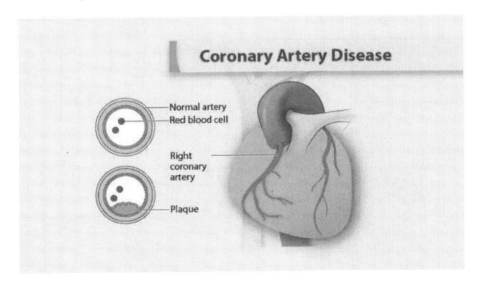

2.3 and above picture source:
https://www.cdc.gov/heartdisease/coronary_ad.htm

2.4 Heart attack

Now that you have an understanding of the heart, coronary artery disease and plaque, let me explain heart attack in simple words here.

1. Plaques form in the artery.

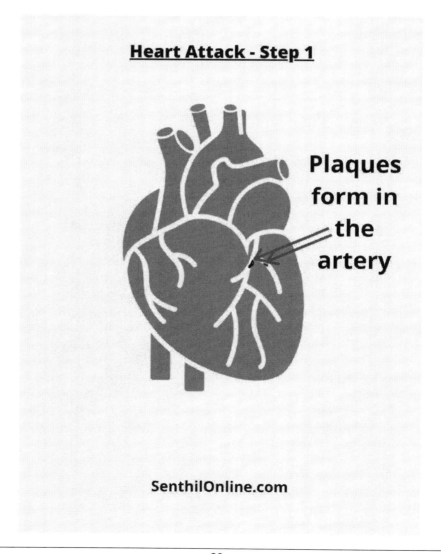

Heart Attack - Step 1

Plaques form in the artery

SenthilOnline.com

2. And one day, these plaques break into smaller pieces.

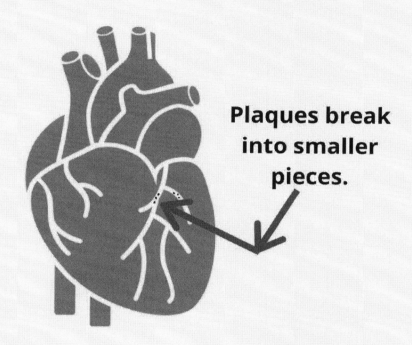

Heart Attack - Step 2

Plaques break into smaller pieces.

SenthilOnline.com

3. Blood starts to clot on these broken plaque pieces and grows, blocking blood flow in the arteries.

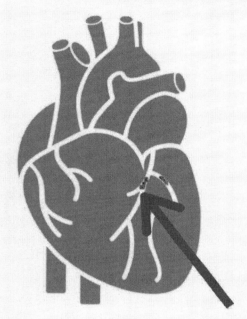

Heart Attack - Step 3

Blood starts to clot on these broken plaque pieces, and grows, blocking blood flow in the arteries.

SenthilOnline.com

4. Because of the blocked arteries, part of the heart muscles does not get Oxygen.

5. The heart muscles that don't get oxygen die. This death of heart muscles is called myocardial infarction or heart attack.

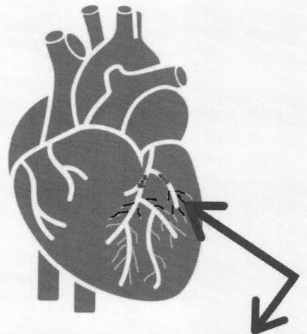

Heart Attack - Step 4 & 5

Part of Heart Muscles that don't get Oxygen, start to die, (shown in black color) causing Heart Attack

SenthilOnline.com

In short, heart attack happens because

1. Plaques form in the artery.

2. And one day, these plaques break into smaller pieces.

3. Blood starts to clot on these broken plaque pieces and grows, blocking blood flow in the arteries.

4. Because of the blocked arteries, part of the heart muscles does not get Oxygen.

5. The heart muscles that don't get oxygen die. This death of heart muscles is called myocardial infarction or heart attack.

2.5 Cardiac Arrest And Heart Failure

2.5.1 Cardiac Arrest

Cardiac arrest is the stopping of the heart. This can happen, if enough of the heart muscles die and the heart stops pumping. The heart has to be revived so that it can start ticking. Otherwise, the person passes away since blood stops flowing to brain and other vital organs.

For more details about heart failure, check NIH's (National Institutes of Health) website:

https://www.nhlbi.nih.gov/health-topics/sudden-cardiac-arrest

2.5.2 Heart Failure

Heart failure happens when the heart is not able to pump enough blood for the body's needs. This is an indicator for a future heart attack or cardiac arrest.

For more details about heart failure, check CDC's (Centers for Disease Control and Prevention) website:

https://www.cdc.gov/heartdisease/heart_failure.htm

2.5.3. Cardiac Arrest Vs Heart Failure

There is an easy way to remember the difference between Cardiac arrest & Heart Failure.

You can compare:

1. Cardiac arrest with an electrical problem of heart and
2. Heart Failure with a plumbing problem of heart!

The following picture, courtesy PulsePoint.org shows this difference in an easy way to understand.

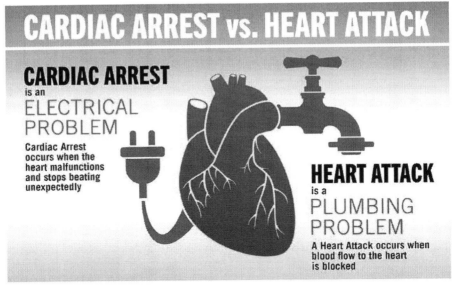

Now you know about heart and various heart diseases.

Next step is to learn how to fix it!

Let us learn the first step to stop attack as part of the 3 Step Formula to "Stop Heart Attack Now!"

References:

Watch the following videos from Khan Academy to understand about Heart Attack, Cardiac Arrest and Heart failure.

Heart Attack (Myocardial Infarct) Diagnosis
https://www.youtube.com/watch?v=T_b9U5gn_Zk

Heart Disease and Heart Attacks
https://www.youtube.com/watch?v=_wre2WRPiFI

3. Step 1 – Know Your Numbers

"Numbers And Letters Are Eyes To All On Earth That Live"

-Thiruvalluvar

Knowing your numbers is very important for your heart health. It can give you a picture of your overall health. And numbers being numbers they don't lie!

Doctors may test for all these numbers when you go for an annual check-up. It is important you know these numbers and understand them.

You should know your:

1. Blood Pressure Numbers
2. Cholesterol Numbers
3. Blood Sugar Number
4. Weight Numbers

Stop Heart Attack Now – Step 1 – Know Your Numbers			
		Normal	
1.	Blood Pressure	Less than 120/80	
2.	Cholesterol	Total <200 LDL < 100	Suggested Target Total 150 Suggested Target LDL < 80 (Read "About Cholesterol Numbers" section below for details)
3.	Blood Sugar (A1c)	Without Diabetes A1c < 5.7% With Diabetes A1c < 7%	
4.	Weight Number - BMI	18.5–24.9	

3.1 Know Your Blood Pressure Numbers

According to National Heart, Lung, and Blood Institute (NHLBI), "High blood pressure is a common condition that is a leading risk factor for heart disease, stroke, and vascular dementia[3.1]." So, to prevent these conditions you should know your blood pressure number.

Following table shows the Normal, Pre-Hypertension and High blood pressure stage 1 and Stage 2 numbers.

Categories for Blood Pressure Levels in Adults
(measured in millimeters of mercury, or mmHg)

Category	Systolic (top number)		Diastolic (bottom number)
Normal	Less than 120	And	Less than 80
Prehypertension	120-139	Or	80-89
High blood pressure			
Stage 1	140-159	Or	90-99
Stage 2	160 or higher	Or	100 or higher

Picture Source:
https://directorsblog.nih.gov/categories-for-blood-pressure/

You might have heard that high blood pressure is called "Silent Killer", because most of the time it shows no sign until it has done significant damage to the heart and arteries.

3.1.2 What To Do If Your Blood Pressure Is High?

Now you know the importance of blood pressure number. If your blood pressure is not normal, you have to take steps to correct this issue. Following are some of the steps you can take per, National Heart, Lung, and Blood Institute (NHLBI)[3.1.2];

1. Eat Healthy Foods
2. Move More
3. Aim for a Healthy Weight
4. Manage Stress
5. Stop Smoking

Eat Healthy Foods

A diet low in sodium and saturated fat—like the DASH eating plan—can lower your blood pressure as effectively as medicines.

1. Add one fruit or vegetable to every meal.
2. If you get fast food, ask for a salad instead fries.
3. Give Meatless Monday a try.
4. Commit to one salt-free day a week. Use herbs for flavor instead.

Move More

Get at least 2½ hours of physical activity a week to help lower and control blood pressure. That's just 30 minutes a day, 5 days a week.

1. Invite a colleague for regular walks or an exercise class.
2. Give the elevator a day off and take the stairs.
3. Take a break to play outside with your kids.
4. March in place during commercial breaks while watching television with your family

Aim for a Healthy Weight

Losing just 3 to 5 percent of your weight can improve your blood pressure. If you weigh 200 lbs., that's a weight loss of 6 to 10 lbs.

1. Join a weight loss program with a buddy.
2. Sign "social support" agreements with three family members or friends

Manage Stress

Stress can contribute to high blood pressure and other heart risks. If it goes on for a long time, it can make your body store more fat.

1. Practice mindful meditation for 10 minutes a day.
2. Share a funny video, joke, or inspirational quote with a friend.
3. Talk with your doctor if you have trouble managing stress on your own

Stop Smoking

The chemicals in tobacco smoke can harm your heart and blood vessels. Quitting is hard. But many people have done it, and you can, too.

1. Visit Smokefree.gov or BeTobaccoFree.hhs.gov to connect with others trying to quit.
2. Sign up for a support group at work or your local clinic.
3. Join a sewing, knitting, or woodworking group to keep your hands busy when you get urges.

Source[3.1]:
https://www.nhlbi.nih.gov/health-topics/education-and-awareness/high-blood-pressure

Source[3.1.2]: Healthy Blood Pressure for Healthy Hearts: Small Steps to Take Control
https://www.nhlbi.nih.gov/sites/default/files/publications/HBP_Infograph_Fact_Sheet_508.pdf

3.2 Know Your Cholesterol Numbers

3.2.1 What Is Cholesterol?

According to cdc.gov, "Blood cholesterol is a waxy, fat-like substance made by your liver. Blood cholesterol is essential for good health. Your body needs it to perform important jobs, such as making hormones and digesting fatty foods.

Your body makes all the blood cholesterol it needs, which is why experts recommend that people eat as little dietary cholesterol as possible while on a healthy eating plan.

Dietary cholesterol is found in animal foods, including meat, seafood, poultry, eggs, and dairy products. Learn more about preventing high cholesterol by making healthy eating choices.

Strong evidence shows that eating patterns that include less dietary cholesterol are associated with reduced risk of cardiovascular disease, but your overall risk depends on many factors."

Source:
https://www.cdc.gov/cholesterol/about.htm

3.2.2 About Cholesterol Numbers - Read this. Very Important

Even though you see the normal total cholesterol number is less than 200 and normal LDL is less than 100 in the image shown in section 3.1 Know Your Numbers Section,

"You have to target total cholesterol levels less than 150 and LDL levels below 80..."

Why?

Reason 1 - NIH Recommendation

Check the Starting Total Cholesterol Number for people over 20 or older, it starts from 125. (I know it says 125 to 200! Read Reason 2)

Healthy Blood Cholesterol Levels, by Age and Sex				
Demographic	Total Cholesterol	Non-HDL	LDL	HDL
Age 19 or younger	Less than 170 mg/dL	Less than 120 mg/dL	Less than 100 mg/dL	More than 45 mg/dL
Men age 20 or older	125 to 200 mg/dL	Less than 130 mg/dL	Less than 100 mg/dL	40 mg/dL or higher
Women age 20 or older	125 to 200 mg/dL	Less than 130 mg/dL	Less than 100 mg/dL	50 mg/dL or higher

Source:
https://www.nhlbi.nih.gov/health-topics/high-blood-cholesterol

Reason 2:

Refer Dr. Caldwell Esselstyn in his book, "Prevent and Reverse Heart Disease" - Page 67. He writes his target LDL levels for his patients:

**"Here, once again, is the basic message of my research: no one who achieves and maintains total blood cholesterol of 150 mg/dl and LDL levels below 80 mg/dl - using strict plant-based nutrition and, where necessary, low doses of cholesterol-reducing drug - experiences progression of heart disease."**

Cholesterol tests are called Lipid Profile or Lipid Panel test. This test normally includes the following:

1. Total Cholesterol
2. Triglycerides
3. HDL Cholesterol
4. LDL Cholesterol
5. Total Cholesterol/HDL Ratio

Cholesterol tests evaluate the risk for developing atherosclerosis (arterial plaque) and coronary heart disease. So, it is very important that you know the cholesterol numbers.

3.3 Know Your Blood Sugar Number

3.3.1 What Is Blood Sugar And Diabetes?

Per cdc.gov, "Most of the food you eat is broken down into sugar (also called glucose) and released into your bloodstream for use as your body's main source of energy.

Diabetes is a condition in which blood sugar levels are too high. If you have type 1 or type 2 diabetes, it is very important to keep your blood sugar numbers in your target range. You may need to check your blood sugar levels several times each day."[3.3.1]

3.3.2 Abnormal Blood Sugar And Cardiovascular Diseases

Is there a link to cardiovascular diseases due to abnormal blood sugar number? Yes. Here is what nih.gov says about this;

"Over time, high blood glucose from diabetes can damage your blood vessels and the nerves that control your heart and blood vessels. The longer you have diabetes, the higher the chances that you will develop heart disease."[3.3.2]

Now you know the importance of blood sugar number. Know this number to prevent heart disease and other diseases mentioned above.

References:

Section[3.3.1]

https://www.cdc.gov/diabetes/managing/manage-blood-sugar.html

Section[3.3.2]

https://www.niddk.nih.gov/health-information/diabetes/overview/preventing-problems/heart-disease-stroke#lower

3.4 Know Your Weight Numbers

According to NHLBI (National Heart, Lung and Blood Institute)[3.4], three key measures are involved in assessment of weight and health risk. They are:

1. Body Mass Index
2. Waist Circumference
3. Risk factors for diseases and conditions associated with obesity

3.4.1 Weight - Body Mass Index (BMI)

Body mass index (BMI) is a measure of body fat based on height and weight that applies to adult men and women.3.4

The following is an excellent write up from nih.gov about BMI.

BMI is a useful measure of overweight and obesity. It is calculated from your height and weight. BMI is an estimate of body fat and a good gauge of your risk for diseases that can occur with more body fat.

The higher your BMI, the higher your risk for certain diseases such as heart disease, high blood pressure, type 2 diabetes, gallstones, breathing problems, and certain cancers.

Although BMI can be used for most men and women, it does have some limits:

It may overestimate body fat in athletes and others who have a muscular build. It may underestimate body fat in older persons and others who have lost muscle.

Use the BMI Calculator or BMI Tables to estimate your body fat. The BMI score means the following:

BMI – Body Mass Index	
Underweight	Below 18.5
Normal	**18.5–24.9**
Overweight	25.0–29.9
Obesity	30.0 and Above

Source:[3.4]
https://www.nhlbi.nih.gov/health/educational/lose_wt/risk.htm

You can calculate your Body Mass Index by visiting the following sites:

1. https://www.nhlbi.nih.gov/health/educati onal/lose_wt/BMI/bmicalc.htm

2. https://www.cdc.gov/healthyweight/asse ssing/bmi/adult_bmi/english_bmi_calcula tor/bmi_calculator.html3.4.1

3.4.2 Know Your Waist Circumference Number

According to CDC.Gov, "Another way to estimate your potential disease risk is to measure your waist circumference.

Excessive abdominal fat may be serious because it places you at greater risk for developing obesity-related conditions, such as Type 2 Diabetes, high blood pressure, and coronary artery disease.

Your waistline may be telling you that you have a higher risk of developing obesity-related conditions if you are:

1. A man whose waist circumference is more than 40 inches

2. A non-pregnant woman whose waist circumference is more than 35 inches

The following picture courtesy cdc.gov shows how to correctly measure the waist circumference.

How To Measure Your Waist Circumference[2]

To correctly measure waist circumference:

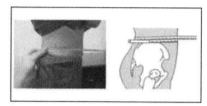

- Stand and place a tape measure around your middle, just above your hipbones
- Make sure tape is horizontal around the waist
- Keep the tape snug around the waist, but not compressing the skin
- Measure your waist just after you breathe out

Waist circumference can be used as a screening tool but is not diagnostic of the body fatness or health of an individual.

A trained healthcare provider should perform appropriate health assessments in order to evaluate an individual's health status and risks."

Source:
https://www.cdc.gov/healthyweight/assessing/index.html

3.4.3 Risk Factors For Diseases And Conditions Associated With Obesity

Per NHLBI (National Heart, Lung and Blood Institute), along with being overweight or obese, the following conditions will put you at greater risk for heart disease and other conditions:

Risk Factors

High blood pressure (hypertension)

High LDL cholesterol ("bad" cholesterol)

Low HDL cholesterol ("good" cholesterol)

High triglycerides

High blood glucose (sugar)

Family history of premature heart disease

Physical inactivity

Cigarette smoking

Source:
https://www.nhlbi.nih.gov/health/educational/lose_wt/risk.htm

Chapter 3 Summary

We are at the end of this chapter. To recap you should know your:

1. Blood Pressure Numbers
2. Cholesterol Numbers
3. Blood Sugar Number
4. Weight Numbers

If your numbers are good. Great! You are in the right direction that can lead you to live a healthy life that can prevent harmful diseases. The next two steps can give you a boost to this goal.

If any of the above numbers are not normal, then nip it in the bud.

Fix it NOW!

Seriously. Don't think this is a minor problem. Do whatever is needed to fix these numbers. By fixing it, you can avert a major disease crisis in your life.

I missed a chance by not fixing my cholesterol numbers early. I don't want this to happen to anyone.

The next two steps can help you achieve normal numbers and can prevent heart disease and other diseases, because heart healthy foods can keep the whole body healthy.

4. Step 2 – Eat Heart Healthy Foods

"__The guidelines for those patients with heart disease are simple:__
__No meat__
__No dairy__
__No oil or nuts__
__Minimal salt and sweetener__
__What can you eat? A delicious and colorful array of vegetables, fruits, legumes, and whole grains, brimming with fiber, nutrients, and antioxidants, all great nourishment for your heart and your overall health."__

__Excerpt from "The Prevent and Reverse Heart Disease Cookbook"__
__Written by: Ann Crile Esselstyn & Jane Esselstyn__

In essence, the step 2 to stop heart attack is to follow No Meat, No Dairy, No Oil or Nuts and Minimal salt and sweetener diet and eat heart healthy foods consisting of vegetables, fruits, legumes and whole grains.

This diet can prevent not only heart diseases but can reverse heart disease!

How cool is that?

This was proven by Dr. Caldwell B. Esselstyn, Jr., MD's research with a group of patients. Check my

Recommended Books section for more details on this.

After reading the above guidelines, I guess your reaction would be one of the following. You may be like:

1."I do not know how to cook without meat, dairy, oil or nuts".

Or

2."No Way... These guidelines are hard. I can't do it!".

If cooking using this guideline is the problem, then fear not! Here is my recommended cookbook - *The Prevent and Reverse Heart Disease Cookbook* to cook awesome meals following these guidelines.

If you think these guidelines are hard, then think again! Would you choose healthy heart and healthy body or surgery? If you consider your wellbeing and your family's wellbeing, I don't think it is hard to switch.

Listed below are some of the heart healthy Vegetables, Fruits, Legumes and Whole grains. This list is not exhaustive and does not cover everything since it is impossible to list them all. The items are listed in no specific order.

Disclosure: I usually take 4 almonds everyday (soaked overnight) and use a minuscule amount of oil in cooking. If you can prepare meals without oil that would be great!

4.1 Eat Vegetables

An article from Agricultural Research Service (ARS), the U.S. Department of Agriculture's (USDA) chief scientific in-house research agency, lists various benefits of Dark green leafy vegetables. Following is a gist of it, in relation to heart health.

"Dark green leafy vegetables are great sources of nutrition. **Salad greens, Kale and Spinach** are rich in vitamins A, C, E and K, and broccoli, bok choy and mustard are also rich in many of the B-vitamins.

The dark greens supply a significant amount of folate, a B vitamin that promotes heart health and helps prevent certain birth defects.

The vitamin K, contents of dark green leafy vegetables provide a number of health benefits including: protecting bones from osteoporosis and helping to **prevent against inflammatory diseases**.

Because of their high content of antioxidants, green leafy vegetables may be one of the best cancer-preventing foods. Studies have shown that eating 2 to 3 servings of green leafy vegetables per week may lower the risk of stomach, breast and skin cancer. These same antioxidants have also been **proven to decrease the risk of heart disease**."

The article also suggests different ways to enjoy leafy green vegetables. We suggest with no meat of course!

Following are few of the ways you can enjoy leafy green vegetables

1. In a Salad
2. Wrap them
3. Add to soup
4. Steamed

Source:
https://www.ars.usda.gov/plains-area/gfnd/gfhnrc/docs/news-2013/dark-green-leafy-vegetables/

4.1.1 Few More Examples of Leafy Green Vegetables

Following are some the leafy green vegetables:

1. Kale
2. Spinach
3. Cabbage
4. Swiss Chard
5. Arugula
6. Collard Greens
7. Beet Greens
8. Mustard Greens
9. Turnip Greens
10. Watercress
11. Romaine Lettuce

Note: If you find Kale is hard to eat, use baby kale which is more tender.

4.1.2 Few More Recommended Vegetables

And following are few more recommended vegetables.

1. Asparagus
2. Tomatoes
3. Squash
4. Bell Peppers
5. Carrots
6. Broccoli
7. Cauliflower
8. Cabbage
9. Celery
10. Zucchini

Apart from the ones listed above, I suggest you to include a mix of other seasonal vegetables in your diet to get maximum health benefits.

4.2 Eat Fruits

"Eating a diet rich in vegetables and fruits as part of an overall healthy diet may reduce risk for heart disease, including heart attack and stroke."

Source:
https://www.choosemyplate.gov/eathealthy/fruits/fruits-nutrients-health

4.2.1 Few Recommended Fruits

Following are a few heart healthy fruits.

1. Berries
   a. Strawberries, Blueberries, Blackberries and Raspberries
2. Red Grapes
3. Tart Cherries
4. Oranges
5. Cantaloupes
6. Papaya

Apart from the above-mentioned fruits, my suggestion is to eat a mix of other fresh fruits such as Apples, Bananas, Pears, Peaches and other seasonal fruits etc. for overall health.

4.2.2 How Much Fruit Is Needed Daily?

The amount of fruit you need to eat depends on age, sex, and level of physical activity. The amount each person needs can vary between 1 and 2 cups each day. Those who are very physically active may need more. Recommended daily amounts are shown in the table below.

Daily Recommendations*		
Children	2-3 yrs	1 cup
	4-8 yrs	1 to 1½ cups
Girls	9-13 yrs	1½ cups
	14-18 yrs	1½ cups
Boys	9-13 yrs	1½ cups
	14-18 yrs	2 cups
Women	19-30 yrs	2 cups
	31-50 yrs	1½ cups
	51+ yrs	1½ cups
Men	19-30 yrs	2 cups
	31-50 yrs	2 cups
	51+ yrs	2 cups

*These amounts are appropriate for individuals who get less than 30 minutes per day of moderate physical activity, beyond normal daily activities. Those who are more physically active may be able to consume more while staying within calorie needs.

Source:
https://www.choosemyplate.gov/eathealthy/fruits

4.2.3 What Counts As A Cup Of Fruit?

Some examples of what counts as a fruit cup is shown below.

	Amount that counts as 1 cup of fruit	Other amounts (count as ½ cup of fruit unless noted)
Apple	½ large (3¼" diameter) 1 small (2¼" diameter) 1 cup, sliced or chopped, raw or cooked	½ cup, sliced or chopped, raw or cooked
Applesauce	1 cup	1 snack container (4oz)
Banana	1 cup, sliced 1 large (8" to 9" long)	1 small (less than 6" long)
Cantaloupe	1 cup, diced or melon balls	1 medium wedge (1/8 of a medium melon)
Grapes	1 cup, whole or cut-up 32 seedless grapes	16 seedless grapes

Source:
https://www.choosemyplate.gov/eathealthy/fruits

4.2.4 Fruit To Avoid If You Have Heart Health Issue

Avocados

Regarding avocados I see conflicting data. I just did a search for "avocado heart" in google. You can see the top two results I got. One for and one against it.

🔒 google.com/search?q=avocado+heart

avocado heart

People also ask

Is Avocado fat bad for your heart?   ⌃

Avocados are high in total **fat**, which may lead you to think that they should be avoided if you're concerned about **your heart** health. But the majority **of the fat in an avocado** is monounsaturated **fat**, which may help lower LDL ("**bad**") cholesterol. Sep 20, 2018

www.brgeneral.org › healthy-lifestyle-blog › september › are-avocados-...
Are Avocados Good for Your Heart? - Baton Rouge General

Search for: Is Avocado fat bad for your heart?

Can avocado cause heart attack?   ⌃

However, new research conducted by Cambridge University suggests that the 'healthy fats' contained in **avocados** and other foods including nuts and fish, **can** increase the risk of **heart disease**. As BBC News points out, eating these foods **can** increase your 'good cholesterol' also known as high-density lipoprotein.

www.joe.ie › fitness-health › research-shows-avocados-can-potentially-i...
Research shows that avocados can potentially increase risk of heart ...

In general, if you have a heart condition, my suggestion would be to avoid avocados. Check the following sources for more information.

Source:
https://www.joe.ie/fitness-health/research-shows-avocados-can-potentially-increase-risk-heart-disease-579155

Source:
http://veganheartdoc.blogspot.com/2014/10/nuts-and-avocadoes.html

4.2.5 Fruit To Avoid, If You Are Taking Blood Thinners

Grapefruit

If you are taking blood thinners, read the medication instructions and label.

In my blood thinner medication, they mentioned "Avoid Grapefruit" while taking this medication.

So please check your medication instructions before eating this fruit.

4.2.6 Juicing– Is It All Right To Juice?

Note that I said, eat the fruit. Not to drink fruit juice! Why? See below FAQ from Dr. Esselstyn's website:

"Do not juice. Fructose separated from fiber is too rapidly absorbed and injurious. You lose the benefits of fiber best obtained by eating the fruit. Chew your food."

Source: https://www.dresselstyn.com/site/faq/

4.3 Eat Legumes

4.3.1 What Is A Legume?

Legumes are dry fruit contained within a pod. According to U.S. Forest Service "Legumes are defined as members of the bean family. This family is large and diverse and contains over 16,000 species."

Source:
https://www.fs.fed.us/wildflowers/ethnobotany/food/legumes.shtml

4.3.2 Examples of legumes

Some of the legumes include:

1. Kidney bean
2. Navy bean
3. Pinto bean
4. Lima bean
5. Mung bean
6. Golden gram
7. Green gram
8. Chickpeas
9. Lentils
10. Peanuts etc.

4.3.3 Why To Consume Legumes?

According to medicineplus, "Beans and legumes are rich in plant protein, fiber, B-vitamins, iron, folate, calcium, potassium, phosphorus, and zinc. Most beans are also low in fat.

Legumes are similar to meat in nutrients, but with lower iron levels and no saturated fats. The high protein in legumes make them a great option in place of meat and dairy products. Vegetarians often substitute legumes for meat.

Legumes are a great source of fiber and may help you have regular bowel movements. Just 1 cup (240 mL) of cooked black beans will give you 15 grams (g) of fiber, which is about half of the recommended daily amount for adults.

Legumes are packed with nutrients. They are low in calories, but make you feel full. The body uses the carbohydrates in legumes slowly, over time, providing steady energy for the body, brain, and nervous system.

Eating more legumes as part of a healthy diet can help lower blood sugar, blood pressure, heart rate, and other heart disease and diabetes risks.

Beans and legumes contain antioxidants that help prevent cell damage and fight disease and aging. The fiber and other nutrients benefit the digestive system, and may even help to prevent digestive cancers."

Source:
https://medlineplus.gov/ency/patientinstructio
ns/000726.htm

4.3.4 List Of Legumes

There are so many types of legumes available. So, it is hard to remember them all. In short, all types of beans, peas, lentils and peanuts are legumes.

Please check the following sites for an exhaustive list of legumes.

1. https://ultimatepaleoguide.com/what-are-legumes-paleo/#list-of-legumes

2. http://www.nourishinteractive.com/health y-living/free-nutrition-articles/120-list-legumes#nutrients-in-legumes

4.4 Eat Whole grains

4.4.1 What are grains?

A grain is a seed from a grass plant. Wheat, Maize, Rice, Barley, Oats, Rye and Sorghum are the seven principle grains grown in the world. Grains are also called cereal grains.

4.4.2 Whole Grains

Grains are divided into 2 subgroups: Whole Grains and Refined Grains.

Whole grains are grains that contain all the three parts of a grain namely the bran, endosperm and germ.

Examples of whole grains include whole-wheat flour, bulgur (cracked wheat), oatmeal, whole cornmeal, and brown rice.

4.4.3 Refined Grains

Refined grains have been milled, a process that removes the bran and germ. This is done to give grains a finer texture and improve their shelf life, but it also removes dietary fiber, iron, and many B vitamins.

Some examples of refined grain products are white flour, de-germed cornmeal, white bread and white rice.

Due to the various health benefits provide by whole grains I suggest eating them only instead of refined grains.

4.4.4 How Whole Grains Help Your Heart?

According to "Effects of whole grains on coronary heart disease risk", a study conducted by NCBI (National Center for Biotechnology Information)

1. "**Whole grain** intake consistently has been associated with **improved cardiovascular disease outcomes**, but also with healthy lifestyles, in large observational studies.

2. Whole grains high in viscous fiber (oats, barley) decrease serum low-density lipoprotein cholesterol and blood pressure and improve glucose and insulin responses.

3. Grains high in insoluble fiber (wheat) moderately lower glucose and blood pressure but also have a prebiotic effect.

4. **Obesity is inversely related to whole grain intake.**"

Source:
https://www.ncbi.nlm.nih.gov/pubmed/208209 54

Also check this article, Whole Grains Help Your Heart

Source: https://www.webmd.com/heart-disease/news/20041229/whole-grains-help-your-heart#1

4.4.5 Daily Grain Table

		Daily recommendation* in ounce-equivalents (oz-equiv)	Daily minimum amount of whole grains in ounce-equivalents (oz-equiv)
Children	2-3 yrs	3 oz-equiv	1½ oz-equiv
	4-8 yrs	5 oz-equiv	2½ oz-equiv
Girls	9-13 yrs	5 oz-equiv	3 oz-equiv
	14-18 yrs	6 oz-equiv	3 oz-equiv
Boys	9-13 yrs	6 oz-equiv	3 oz-equiv
	14-18 yrs	8 oz-equiv	4 oz-equiv
Women	19-30 yrs	6 oz-equiv	3 oz-equiv
	31-50 yrs	6 oz-equiv	3 oz-equiv
	51+ yrs	5 oz-equiv	3 oz-equiv
Men	19-30 yrs	8 oz-equiv	4 oz-equiv
	31-50 yrs	7 oz-equiv	3½ oz-equiv
	51+ yrs	6 oz-equiv	3 oz-equiv

*These amounts are appropriate for individuals who get less than 30 minutes per day of moderate physical activity, beyond normal daily activities.

Those who are more physically active may be able to consume more while staying within calorie needs.

Source: https://www.choosemyplate.gov/eathealthy/grains

4.4.6 What counts as an ounce-equivalent of grains?

In general, 1 slice of bread, 1 cup of ready-to-eat cereal, or ½ cup of cooked rice, cooked pasta, or cooked cereal can be considered as 1 ounce-equivalent from the Grains Group.

The following 2 tables below lists specific amounts that count as 1 ounce-equivalent of grains towards your daily recommended intake. In some cases, the number of ounce-equivalents for common portions are also shown.

Table 1

		Amount that counts as 1 ounce-equivalents (oz-equiv) of grains	Common portions and ounce-equivalents (oz-equiv)
Bagels	WG**: whole wheat	1" mini bagel	1 large bagel = 4 oz-equiv
Breads	WG**: 100% Whole Wheat	1 regular slice	2 regular slices = 2 oz-equiv
Bulgur	cracked wheat (WG**)	½ cup, cooked	
Crackers	WG**: 100% whole wheat, rye	5 whole wheat crackers 2 rye crisp breads	
English muffins	WG**: whole wheat	½ muffin	1 muffin = 2 oz-equiv
Muffins	WG**: whole wheat	1 small (2½" diameter)	1 large (3½" diameter) = 3 oz-

*WG = whole grains

Source:
https://www.choosemyplate.gov/eathealthy/grains

Table 2

		Amount that counts as 1 ounce-equivalents (oz-equiv) of grains	Common portions and ounce-equivalents (oz-equiv)
Oatmeal	(WG**)	½ cup, cooked 1 packet instant 1 ounce (⅓ cup), dry (regular or quick)	
Pancakes	WG**: Whole wheat, buckwheat	1 pancake (4½" diameter)	3 pancakes (4½" diameter) = 3 oz-equiv
Popcorn	(WG**)	3 cups, popped	1 mini microwave bag or 100-calorie bag, popped = 2 oz-equiv
Ready-to-eat breakfast cereal	WG**: toasted oat, whole wheat flakes	1 cup, flakes or rounds	
Rice	WG*: brown, wild	½ cup cooked	1 cup, cooked = 2 oz-equiv
Pasta-- spaghetti, macaroni, noodles	WG**: whole wheat	½ cup, cooked	1 cup, cooked = 2 oz-equiv
Tortillas	WG**: whole wheat, whole grain corn	1 small flour tortilla (6" diameter)	1 large tortilla (12" diameter) = 4 oz-equiv

*WG = whole grains

Source:
https://www.choosemyplate.gov/eathealthy/grains

Chapter 4 Summary

In step 2, you know what good foods you have to eat for a healthy heart and body. If you are an inexperienced or experienced cook and wondering how you are going whip a heart healthy breakfast, lunch or dinner using vegetables, legumes and whole grains...Fear not!

Help is in the **Recommended Books** section. All the books that I recommend have a section especially for making nice dishes using healthy produce and more.

And one book in particular namely "**The Prevent and Reverse Heart Disease Cookbook**" has "Over 125 Delicious, Life-Changing, Plant-Based Recipes". So, with all this help you get from these books, you can make heart healthy and tasty breakfasts, lunches, soups, salads, dinners and even desserts too!

If step 2 of "Stop Heart Attack Now" is about feeding the right food to the body, step 3 is about feeding the right content to the brain. Let's head over to step 3.

5.Step 3 – Educate Yourself on Heart Health

"Give a man a fish and you feed him for a day; teach a man to fish and you feed him for a lifetime."

-Proverb

In Step 1 and Step 2 I was telling you what you should do. Step 3 needs your involvement. It is you educating yourself on heart health.

The sub-title of this book says, step 3 is optional. If you don't want to educate yourself on heart health, yes, this step 3 is optional.

Otherwise do not skip this step and **Educate yourself on heart health!**

How can you do this?

5.1 Resources to Educate Yourself on Heart Health

1. Read the books I recommend from the Recommended Books section and update yourself. The authors have vast experience in their respective fields. Learn from them and use it for improving your heart health.

2. Go through all the links and sources in the Links and References section. Gain wealth of knowledge from this section.

Conclusion

If you are reading this, then Congratulations! You did it!

Hope you have a good understanding of the using the 3-step formula now. In summary, to stop heart attack and to reverse heart disease, follow the 3-step formula.

1. Step 1 - Know your numbers

2. Step 2 - Switch to, no meat, no dairy, no oil or nuts and minimal salt and sweetener guidelines and eat heart healthy foods consisting of fruits, vegetables, legumes and whole grains.

3. Step 3 - Educate yourself on heart health.

The next step is implementation! Apply the 3-step formula to stop heart attack and have a healthy heart and healthy body.

Do you know what I would consider as my success in writing this book?

If you apply the 3-step formula and have a healthy heart and healthy body, then, that is success for me!

Pass on a copy of this book "Stop Heart Attack Now" to your family and friends, if you care for their heart and health.

The link to purchase this book is:
http://www.stopheartattacknow.com/

Wishing you good health and happiness...

Senthil Natarajan

Acknowledgments

There are many thanks I'd like to express, to:

Dr. Rajiv K. Aggarwal, MD my primary care physician for immediately diagnosing and referring me to my cardiologist when I suffered from heart attack and to his support

Dr. Ather Anis, MD, my cardiologist for performing angioplasty on me and guiding me on my recovery

Doctors, Nurses, Lab Technicians, Management and other members of Inova Loudoun Hospital, you have an excellent facility for heartcare!

Louise Ann Jones, NP for suggesting me to switch to brown rice and to your support during my regular checkups

All my friends and family members who visited, supported and prayed for my wellbeing during my hospital stay and after

CDC (Centers for Disease Control and Prevention), National Institutes of Health (NIH), National Heart, Lung, and Blood Institute (NHLBI), MedLinePlus.gov, ChooseMyPlate.gov, Agricultural Research Service (ARS) the U.S. Department of Agriculture's (USDA) chief scientific in-house research agency and other government agencies who provide a wealth of health and safety information for the public to use. I have referred and used relevant material from your websites!

Dr.Caldwell B. Esselstyn, Jr., M.D to your excellent book "Prevent and Reverse Heart Disease" and permitting me to use an excerpt from the book and from your website

Ann Crile Esselstyn for your blessing and supporting words

Jane Esselstyn for providing permission to use an excerpt from the "Prevent and Reverse Heart Disease Cookbook". Read this cookbook, if you don't know how to cook plant-based recipes!

All my friends and family members who signed up for this book pre-release and encouraged me and anyone I missed to acknowledge

Finally, to my wife and son...you both stood with me during my heart attack and after... (no words to express.)

A Big Thanks to all of you, from the bottom of my heart!

Reader's Suggestion

What else could I add in this book to stop heart attack?

Please send your suggestions to
senthil@senthilonline.com

I might include it in the next edition of this book!

Brown Rice

Since using brown rice helped in reducing my triglycerides, I have a special place in my heart for it. My research showed it provides various other benefits also. Let us see more about this whole grain in this chapter.

Brown rice has Vitamin B-1 (Thiamin) which can help you protect the heart from the disease called beriberi. Beriberi, is caused by vitamin B-1 deficiency.

According to 24mantra.com "**Brown rice is known to stimulate better functioning of cardiovascular system, digestive system, brain and nervous system**"

And following are some of the health benefits of brown rice listed by them.

1. Rich in Selenium
2. High in Manganese
3. Rich in Naturally Occurring Oils
4. Helps in Weight Loss and more...

Source:
http://www.24mantra.com/whitericevsbrownrice/

Also watch:

"The Truth about Rice... White Rice vs. Brown Rice!"
https://youtu.be/csmkS5GwsWw

I use 24mantra Sonamasuri Organic Brown Rice. I cook it on the stove top and drain the water.

Raw - 24mantra Sonamasuri Organic Brown Rice

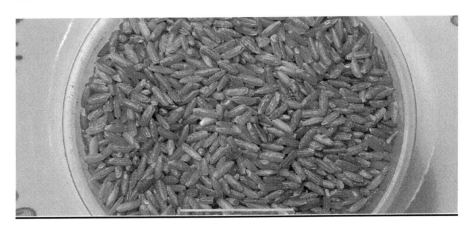

Cooked - 24mantra Sonamasuri Organic Brown Rice

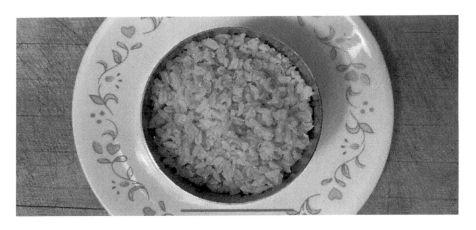

Check my review about this brown rice at:

https://www.senthilonline.com/brown-rice-amzn

Recommended Books

Following are few of my recommended books. Read these books for your heart health and for your wellbeing.

1. Prevent and Reverse Heart Disease: The Revolutionary, Scientifically Proven, Nutrition-Based Cure by Caldwell B. Esselstyn Jr.

2. The Prevent and Reverse Heart Disease Cookbook: Over 125 Delicious, Life-Changing, Plant-Based Recipes – by Ann Crile Esselstyn, Jane Esselstyn

3. Undo It!: How Simple Lifestyle Changes Can Reverse Most Chronic Diseases Hardcover – by Dean Ornish M.D., Anne Ornish

4. The End of Heart Disease: The Eat to Live Plan to Prevent and Reverse Heart Disease - by Joel Fuhrman M.D.

Check my reviews on Heart Health Books in my website.

https://www.senthilonline.com/heart-health-books/

Recommended Products

Standing Desk

According to the Centers of Disease Control and Prevention (CDC):

"Prolonged sitting time (as a specific instance of sedentary behavior), independent of physical activity, has emerged as a risk factor for various negative health outcomes.

Study results have demonstrated associations of prolonged sitting time with premature mortality; chronic diseases such as cardiovascular disease, diabetes, and cancer; metabolic syndrome; and obesity.

In contrast, breaks in prolonged sitting time have been correlated with beneficial metabolic profiles among adults, suggesting that frequent breaks in sedentary activity may explain lower health risk related to waist circumference, body mass index (BMI), triglyceride levels, and 2-hour plasma glucose levels."

Their findings suggest that "using a sit-stand device at work can reduce sitting time and generate other health benefits for workers".

Source: Reducing Occupational Sitting Time and Improving Worker Health: The Take-a-Stand Project, 2011

https://www.cdc.gov/pcd/issues/2012/11_032
3.htm

Also check the following website where they list of many benefits of standing up, sitting less and moving more.

https://www.juststand.org/the-facts/

Standing desk – Do It Yourself

If you have budget constraints to buy a high-ticket standing desk, check the following:

"The Complete Guide to DIY Standing Desks"

https://www.startstanding.org/standing-desks/the-complete-guide-to-diy-standing-desks/#standing

My Webpage on Standing Desks

If you want check few other types of standing desks and for low priced standing desks, check my webpage on Standing Desks

https://www.senthilonline.com/standing-desks/

Links and References

Your FREE Bonus

https://www.senthilonline.com/FREE/

Introduction

Source[1]:

https://www.cdc.gov/heartdisease/facts.htm

Source[2]: Prevent and Reverse Heart Disease by Caldwell B. Esselstyn, Jr., MD – Various angiograms on Reversal of Coronary Disease.

1.My Story

1.1 Day of Attack

1.1.1 What is ECG or EKG

Source:

https://www.webmd.com/heart-disease/electrocardiogram-ekgs#1

1.2 My Angioplasty Experience

https://www.mayoclinic.org/tests-procedures/coronary-angioplasty/multimedia/coronary-angioplasty/vid-20084728

https://www.youtube.com/watch?v=S9AqBd4R
Exk

1.2.1 What Is Angioplasty and Stenting?

1.2.2 Stent

1.2.3 Details About My Angioplasty

1.3 Challenges After Discharge

1.3.1 How to overcome groin pain when lying flat?

1.3.2 How to get to sleep with groin pain?

1.3.1 Isha Chants App Links

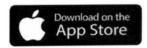

https://apps.apple.com/us/app/isha-
chants/id1158670101

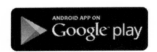

https://play.google.com/store/apps/details?id
=org.ishafoundation.app.chants&hl=en_US

1.4 Lifestyle Change - My Eureka Moment!

1.4.1 What are triglycerides?

Source:

https://medlineplus.gov/triglycerides.html

2.What is a Heart Attack?

2.1 Heart

2.2 What is plaque?

Source:

https://www.cdc.gov/heartdisease/facts.htm

2.3 What is coronary artery disease?

https://www.cdc.gov/heartdisease/coronary_a
d.htm

2.3.1 What causes coronary artery disease?

https://www.cdc.gov/heartdisease/coronary_a
d.htm

2.4 Heart Attack

2.5 Cardiac Arrest and Heart Failure

2.5.1 Cardiac arrest

https://www.nhlbi.nih.gov/health-
topics/sudden-cardiac-arrest

2.5.2 Heart Failure

https://www.cdc.gov/heartdisease/heart_failur
e.htm

3. Step 1 – Know Your Numbers

3.1 Know Your Blood Pressure Numbers

Picture Source:

https://directorsblog.nih.gov/categories-for-blood-pressure/

3.1.2 What to do if your blood pressure is high?

Source: Healthy Blood Pressure for Healthy Hearts: Small Steps to Take Control

https://www.nhlbi.nih.gov/sites/default/files/publications/HBP_Infograph_Fact_Sheet_508.pdf

3.2 Know Your Cholesterol Numbers

Source:

https://www.nhlbi.nih.gov/health-topics/education-and-awareness/high-blood-pressure

3.2.1 What is Cholesterol?

Source:

https://www.cdc.gov/cholesterol/about.htm

3.2.2 About Cholesterol Numbers - Read this. Very Important

Source:

https://www.nhlbi.nih.gov/health-topics/high-blood-cholesterol

3.3 Know Your Blood Sugar Number
3.3.1 What Is Blood Sugar and Diabetes?

https://www.cdc.gov/diabetes/managing/manage-blood-sugar.html

3.3.2 Abnormal Blood Sugar and Cardiovascular Diseases

https://www.niddk.nih.gov/health-information/diabetes/overview/preventing-problems/heart-disease-stroke#lower

3.4 Know Your Weight Numbers
Source[1]:

https://www.nhlbi.nih.gov/health/educational/lose_wt/risk.htm

3.4.1 Weight - Body Mass Index (BMI)
You can calculate your Body Mass Index by visiting the following sites:

https://www.nhlbi.nih.gov/health/educational/lose_wt/BMI/bmicalc.htm

https://www.cdc.gov/healthyweight/assessing/bmi/adult_bmi/english_bmi_calculator/bmi_calculator.html

3.4.2 Know Your Waist Circumference Number

Source:

https://www.cdc.gov/healthyweight/assessing/index.html

3.4.3 Risk factors for diseases and conditions associated with obesity

Source:

https://www.nhlbi.nih.gov/health/educational/lose_wt/risk.htm

Chapter 3 Summary

4. Step 2 – Eat Heart Healthy Foods

4.1 Eat Vegetables

Source:

https://www.ars.usda.gov/plains-area/gfnd/gfhnrc/docs/news-2013/dark-green-leafy-vegetables/

4.1.1 Few More Examples of Leafy Green Vegetables

4.1.2 Few More Recommended Vegetables

4.2 Eat Fruits

Source:

https://www.choosemyplate.gov/eathealthy/fruits/fruits-nutrients-health

4.2.1 Few Recommended Fruits

4.2.2 How much fruit is needed daily?

Source:

https://www.choosemyplate.gov/eathealthy/fruits

4.2.3 What counts as a cup of fruit?

Source:

https://www.choosemyplate.gov/eathealthy/fruits

4.2.2 Fruit to Avoid If You Have Heart Health Issue

Source:

https://www.joe.ie/fitness-health/research-shows-avocados-can-potentially-increase-risk-heart-disease-579155

Source:

http://veganheartdoc.blogspot.com/2014/10/nuts-and-avocadoes.html

4.2.3 Fruit to Avoid, If You Are Taking Blood Thinners.

4.2.3 Juicing– Is it all right to juice?

Source: https://www.dresselstyn.com/site/faq/

4.3 Eat Legumes

4.3.1 What is a legume?

Source:

https://www.fs.fed.us/wildflowers/ethnobotany/food/legumes.shtml

4.3.2 Examples of legumes

4.3.3 Why to consume legumes?

Source:

https://medlineplus.gov/ency/patientinstructions/000726.htm

4.3.4 List of Legumes

4.4 Eat Whole grains

4.4.1 What are grains?

4.4.2 Whole grains (WG)

4.4.2 Refined grains (RG)

4.4.3 How Whole Grains Help Your Heart?

Source:

https://www.ncbi.nlm.nih.gov/pubmed/20820954

Source:

https://www.webmd.com/heart-disease/news/20041229/whole-grains-help-your-heart#1

4.4.4 Daily Grain Table

Source:

https://www.choosemyplate.gov/eathealthy/grains

4.4.5 What counts as an ounce-equivalent of grains?

Source:

https://www.choosemyplate.gov/eathealthy/grains

Chapter 4 Summary

5.Step 3 – Educate Yourself on Heart Health

5.1 Resources to Educate Yourself on Heart Health

Conclusion

Reader's Suggestion

Brown Rice

24mantra Sonamasuri Organic Brown Rice
Source:
http://www.24mantra.com/whitericevsbrownri
ce/

"The Truth about Rice... White Rice vs. Brown Rice!"
https://youtu.be/csmkS5GwsWw

Check my review about this brown rice at:
https://www.senthilonline.com/brown-rice-
amzn

Recommended Products

Standing Desk

Source: Reducing Occupational Sitting Time and Improving Worker Health: The Take-a-Stand Project, 2011
https://www.cdc.gov/pcd/issues/2012/11_0323.htm

Also check the following website. In this website, they list out many benefits of standing up, sitting less and moving more.
https://www.juststand.org/the-facts/

Standing desk – Do It Yourself

If you have budget constraints to buy a high-ticket standing desk, check the following:
"The Complete Guide to DIY Standing Desks"

My Webpage on Standing Desks

If you want check few other types of standing desks and for low priced standing desks, check my webpage on Standing Desks

https://www.senthilonline.com/standing-desks/

Recommended Books

1. Prevent and Reverse Heart Disease: The Revolutionary, Scientifically Proven, Nutrition-Based Cure by Caldwell B. Esselstyn Jr.

2. The Prevent and Reverse Heart Disease Cookbook: Over 125 Delicious, Life-Changing, Plant-Based Recipes – by Ann Crile Esselstyn, Jane Esselstyn

3. Undo It!: How Simple Lifestyle Changes Can Reverse Most Chronic Diseases Hardcover – by Dean Ornish M.D., Anne Ornish

4. The End of Heart Disease: The Eat to Live Plan to Prevent and Reverse Heart Disease - by Joel Fuhrman M.D.

Check my reviews on Heart Health Books in my website.

https://www.senthilonline.com/heart-health-books/

About the Author

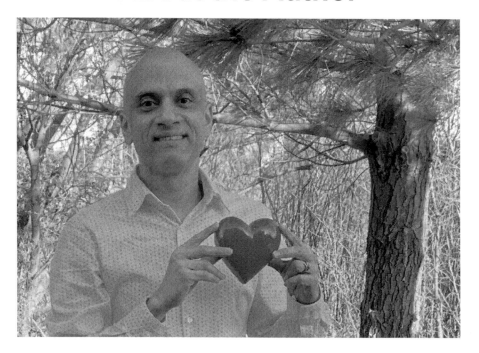

Senthil Natarajan is an information technology (IT) professional. After his heart attack a few years ago, he devoted more attention to his heart health and to his overall wellbeing. Now, he wants to share his learnings about heart health, heart attack recovery and wellbeing with others.

Every time he learns someone has a heart incidence, he feels it need not happen that way and they could have prevented it, by taking simple steps to prevent a heart attack from happening.

This book and its 3 steps formula are the result of that urge, so people can use this information and prevent heart disease and heart related issues.

Stay connected with him for his future releases, updates etc.

Subscribe to his email list.

You also get a Heart Healthy Drinks Series as FREE BONUS! when you signup...

https://www.senthilonline.com/FREE/

Connect with me on twitter
https://twitter.com/nsenthilonline

Do you have a heart attack or heart disease recovery success story to share? Get in touch and you may be featured in a future version of this book!
https://www.senthilonline.com/contact/

Thank You!

"Thank You" for purchasing this book and reading all the way to the end.

Hopefully you got a better understanding what to do for heart health now and learnt the 3-step formula to stop the heart attack. Heart healthy foods can help in your overall health also.

<u>Please take a minute, to leave me a quick review on Amazon.</u>

To write a review visit:
http://www.StopHeartAttackNow.com/

<u>Your feedback is important and valuable because it can guide the future editions of this book.</u>

<u>Thanks in advance for your help!</u>

Made in the USA
Columbia, SC
08 May 2020

96574799R00064